This book belongs to:

_____

Children Who Eat Their Fruits and Vegetables

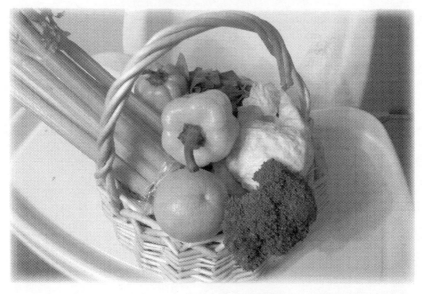

MORE VEGGIES PLEASE!

Philomina U. Emeka-Iheukwu

iUniverse, Inc.
Bloomington

CHILDREN WHO EAT THEIR FRUITS AND VEGETABLES

iUniverse books may be ordered through booksellers or by contacting:

iUniverse
1663 Liberty Drive
Bloomington, IN 47403
www.iuniverse.com
1-800-Authors (1-800-288-4677)

ISBN: 978-1-4759-7736-3 (sc)
ISBN: 978-1-4759-7737-0 (e)

Printed in the United States of America

iUniverse rev. date: 2/22/2013

To my original children, Sylvester and Sabella; Chelsea, my niece who is so dear to my heart, Somtochukwu; my very handsome nephew, Somkenechukwu; my very own beautiful cousin I'm yet to meet but very close to my heart. To Emmanuella, Sylvan, Bonnie and Paris McGhee; my precious nieces and nephew, and to all the children around the world

Cherish what keeps you nourished;

Cherish what keeps you nourished.

Go for it and never give up;

You will give your energy a boost,

And you will be glad you did at last.

Cherish what keeps you nourished.

Sylvester and Sabella love their fruits and vegetables. They ate vegetables all day long and couldn't get enough of it. It really showed as they were lean and fit, strong and healthy. Everyone gave them a credit for it. Three years in a row, they had won the school kids' vegetable contest held annually to encourage healthy eating. They love their vegetables very much.

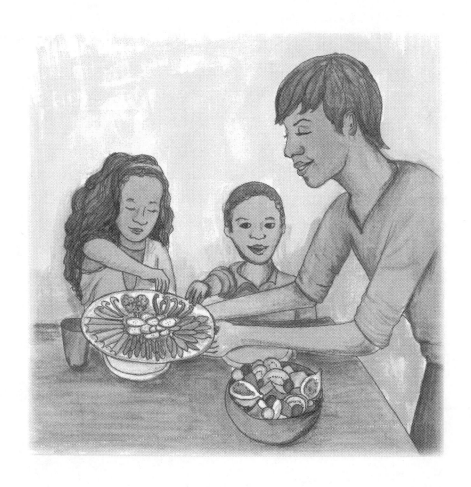

It was a summer Saturday morning, one that Sabella was long waiting for. It was their visiting day to their best friend's, Chelsea Emeka. The twins and Chelsea were friends right from the womb, their mothers had met on one of those prenatal visits and remained close friends ever since. The kids nearly shared the same age; but the twins were only five months older than Chelsea. Chelsea and her friends almost had everything in common but one thing and one thing only- VEGETABLES- Chelsea was very picky and her mother worried if her friends could help do the trick. She had tried several times, but nothing had changed; at all. The day before, Mrs. Emeka had gone grocery shopping. Her refrigerator was filled to the brim with the healthiest foods ever, fruits and vegetables of course!

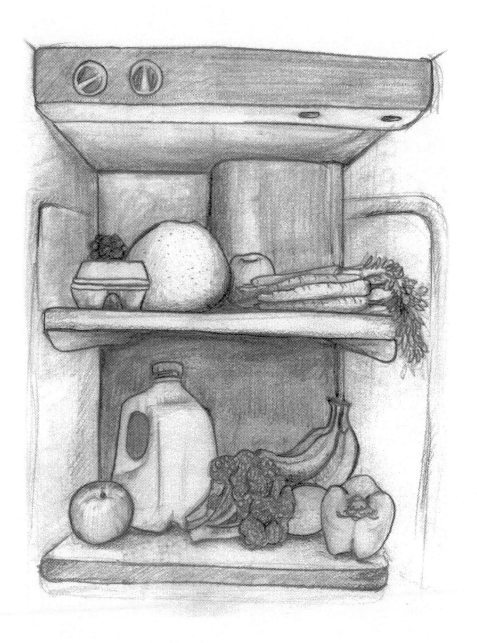

She hoped her child might like to try at least one during the vegetable party. She was a bit nervous as they waited for their guests to arrive. Soon, the doorbell rang; 'tilum... tilum...'

Mrs. Emeka and her daughter went to get the door and standing before them were their long awaited friends.

"Hello Uzo, welcome!" Mrs. Emeka greeted, opening the door wider to let them in. "This is for you," Uzo said, offering a bouquet of beautiful flowers to her friend.

"Oh, these are beautiful! How nice of you? Well, thank you." she greeted, admiring the flowers and then put them in a vase right away.

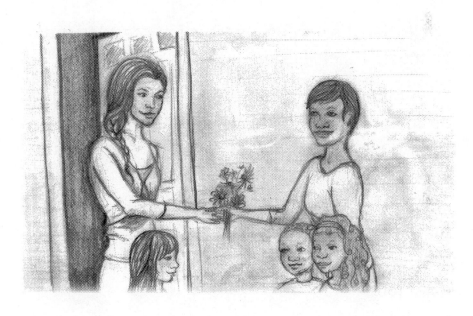

"Hello Sabella, Hello Sylvester, I missed you guys so much." Chelsea said, hugging her friends.

"Same here, we greatly missed you too," they admitted. Chelsea took her friends to her playhouse while the ladies got the table ready for the big vegetable party.

The table was set with lots and lots of colorful fruits and vegetables. The arrangement was attractive and appetizing; the women did a very good job.

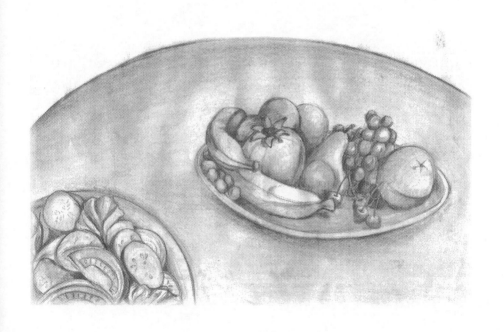

They finally covered the table with beautiful pink lace. Pink was Chelsea's favorite color, but nobody knows if she would like to try what was hidden under her favorite pink lace.

"Come on kids! It's time for our lunch party." Mrs. Emeka called nervously, she didn't know what to expect.

"Alright!" they replied running excitedly to the dining-room.

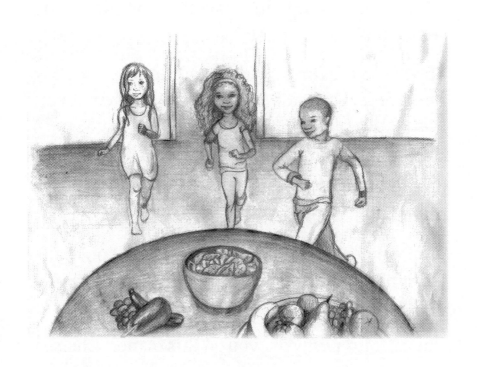

"This is beautiful lace!" Sabella said remarkably.

"That's my favorite!" Chelsea admitted, feeling the lace as she sat herself down. Everyone was seated but Chelsea's mum.

"Chelsea darling," she began. "This is going to be a lot of fun." she said, sliding the lace away to reveal their secret.

"Cool veggies!" exclaimed the twins. "Look how colorful they are!" Sabella added, encouraging her friend to try.

"Eww... Mum, why did you do this to me?" Chelsea cried.

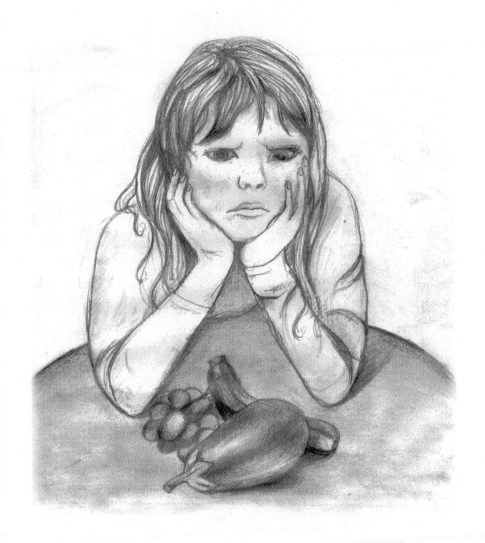

"Your mother only wants you to be healthy." Uzo said nicely.

"Come on, Chelsea, you can do this." the twins said, almost at the same time.

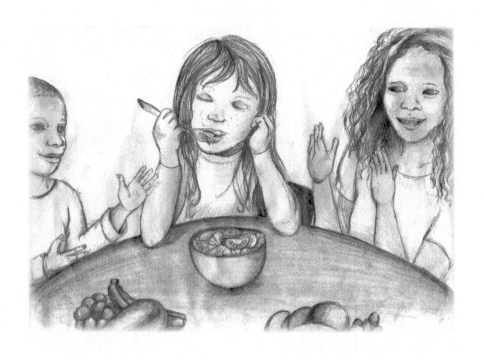

Sabella then offered her a piece of carrot. Chelsea loves her friend so much and finds it extremely difficult to resist her plea. She was about to try some food, and then suddenly changed her mind.

"This is going to be difficult," Chelsea complained then took a deep breath.

"How could you tell if you don't try?" Sabella asked politely.

"I will try...e...emm...em...only if you can guess which one is on my mind," she said.

"That's easy; we know our fruits and vegetables! Sylvester exclaimed innocently not imaging how tough that could be.

Then they began and the mothers cheered not knowing what to expect still.

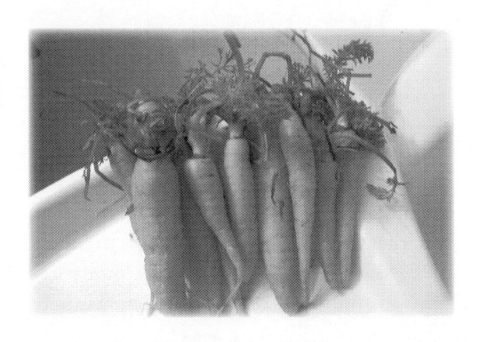

"Eat your carrots. Yum, yum, yum;

Carrots surely are yum, yum, yum;

Carrots are crunchy and delicious;

Carrots surely are good for you.

Vitamins and Minerals are good for you;

Good for your eyes, good for your skin;

Good for your heart, teeth and gums.

Eat your carrots daily. Yum, yum, yum!"

They chanted and chanted to have her try. Chelsea nodded in disapproval then chanted back:

"No thank you! It's not that one.

Try again, it's not that one."

Cheerers looked at one another then tried Broccoli.

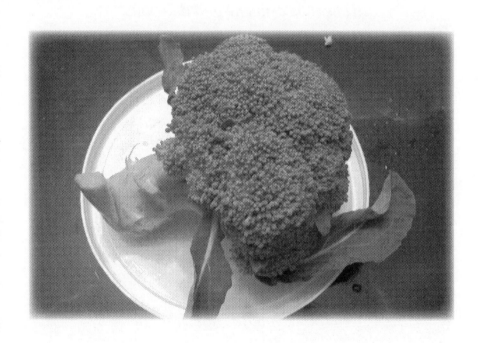

"Eat your broccoli. Yum, yum, yum;

Broccoli surely is yum, yum, yum;

Broccoli is crunchy and delicious;

Broccoli surely is good for you.

Vitamins and Minerals are good for you;

Good for your eyes, good for your skin;

Good for your heart, muscles and bones.

Eat your broccoli daily, yum, yum, yum!"

They chanted and cheered to have her try. Chelsea shook her head in disapproval then chanted back:

"No thank you! It's not that one.

Try again, it's not that one."

Everyone looked at one another then tried Onions.

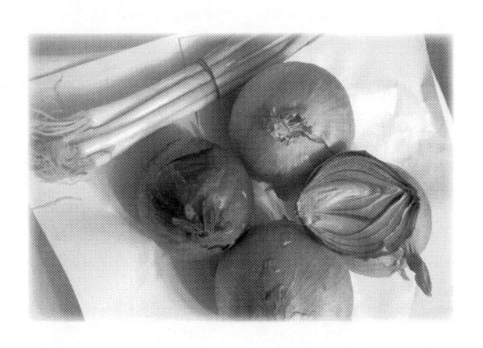

"Eat your onions. Yum, yum, yum;

Onions surely are yum, yum, yum;

Onions are crunchy and delicious;

Onions surely are good for you.

Vitamins and Minerals are good for you;

Good for your hair, good for your skin;

Good for your heart, soothes colds and flu.

Eat your onions, yum, yum, yum!"

They chanted and chanted to have her try. Chelsea shook her head in disapproval then replied.

"No thank you! It's not that one.

Try again, it's not that one."

She was really enjoying her trick but chanters were still very strong and decided they would try Kale.

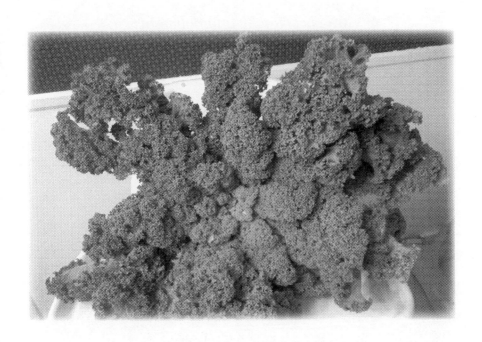

"Eat your kale. Yum, yum, yum;

Kale surely is yum, yum, yum;

Kale is crunchy and delicious;

Kale surely is good for you.

Vitamins and Minerals are good for you;

Good for your blood, good for your bones;

Good for your heart; high in fiber too.

Eat your kale daily, yum, yum, yum!"

They cheered to have her try. Chelsea chuckled, shook her head in disapproval then chanted so:

"No thank you! It's not that one.

Try yet another, it's not that one."

Chanters looked at one another then chose Cucumbers.

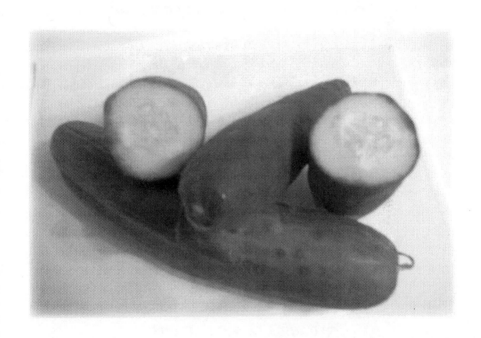

"Eat your cucumbers. Yum, yum, yum;

Cucumbers surely are yum, yum, yum;

Cucumbers are crunchy and delicious;

Cucumbers surely are good for you.

Vitamins and Minerals are good for you;

Good for your hair, nails, tummy and skin;

Good for your joints, weight, teeth and gums.

Eat cucumbers daily, yum, yum, yum!"

They chanted and cheered to have her try. Chelsea shook her head then chanted back:

"No thank you! It's not that one.

Try again, it's not that one."

Chanters thought and thought then wondered why they haven't being able to guess it right. They made a decision and it was Peppers.

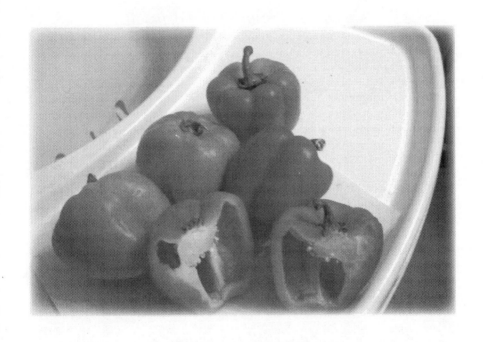

"Eat your peppers. Yum, yum, yum;

Peppers surely are yum, yum, yum;

Peppers are crunchy and delicious;

Peppers surely are good for you.

Vitamins and Minerals are good for you;

Good for your eyes, cells, bones and skin;

Good for your heart, high in fiber too.

Eat your peppers daily. Yum, yum, yum!"

They chanted and cheered to have her try. Chelsea chuckled, shook her head then chanted again:

"No thank you! It's not that one.

Try again, it's not that one."

Chanters yet looked at one another and decided it must be Cabbage.

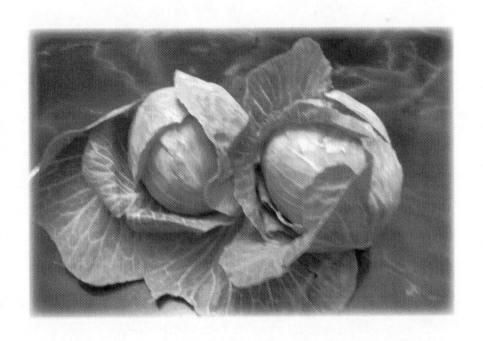

"Eat your cabbage. Yum, yum, yum;

Cabbage surly is yum, yum, yum;

Cabbage is crunchy and delicious;

Cabbage surely is good for you.

Vitamins and Minerals are good for you;

Good for your eyes, brains, bones and skin;

Good for your heart, weight, tummy and hair.

Eat your cabbage; it is yum, yum, yum!"

They chanted and cheered to have her try. Chelsea shook her head from left to right.

"No thank you! It's not that one

Try another one! It's not that one."

Chanters were getting exhausted. Uzo went to rest but others have to try. This time around, they chose Brussels sprouts.

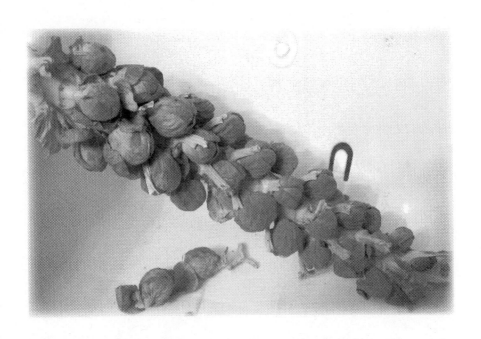

"Eat Brussels sprouts. Yum, yum, yum;

Brussels sprouts surely are yum, yum, yum;

Brussels sprouts are crunchy and delicious;

Brussels sprouts surely are good for you.

Vitamins and Minerals are good for you;

Good for your eyes, cells, bones and brains;

Good for your heart, liver, tummy, teeth and fiber too.

Eat your Brussels sprouts; yum, yum, yum!"

They did all they could to have her try but Chelsea shook her head again and again.

"No thank you! It's not that one.

You just have to try, it's not that one."

Chanters made a decision and then picked Beets.

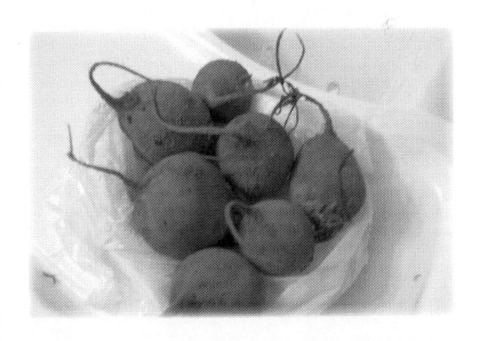

"Eat your beets. They are yum, yum, yum;

Beets surely are yum, yum, yum;

Beets are crispy and delicious;

Beets surely are good for you.

Vitamins and Minerals are good for you;

Good for your blood, cells and bones;

Good for your heart, liver, weight and fiber too.

Eat beets daily. Beets are yum, yum, yum!"

They cheered even louder to have her try but Chelsea shook her head no, no, no.

"No thank you! It's not that one.

Try and try, it's not that one."

Sylvester got exhausted then went to rest. Only two were left to chant and cheer. They put their heads together and then made a decision. It was Spinach.

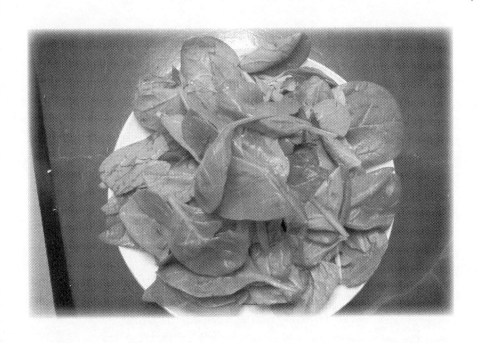

"Eat your Spinach. Yum, yum, yum;

Spinach surely is yum, yum, yum;

Spinach is crispy and delicious;

Spinach surely is good for you.

Vitamins and Minerals are good for you;

Good for your eyes, cells, bones, brains and skin;

Good for your heart, tummy, blood and fiber too.

Eat spinach daily, it is yum, yum, yum!"

They cheered and cheered to have her try; but Chelsea shook her head and laughed at them.

"No thank you! It's not that one.

You may try again, not that one."

They made another choice and it was Eggplant.

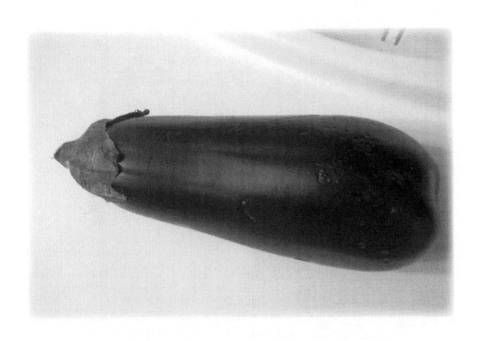

"Eat your eggplant. Yum, yum, yum;

Eggplant surely is yum, yum, yum;

Eggplant is crispy and delicious;

Eggplant surely is good for you.

Vitamins and Minerals are good for you;

Good for your hair, cells, brains and skin;

Good for your heart, tummy and high fiber too.

Eat eggplants daily. Yum, yum, yum!"

They chanted and cheered to have her try; Chelsea still shook her head in disapproval and then chanted back:

"No thank you! It's not that one.

Try again. It's not that one."

They then made a choice and it was Lettuce.

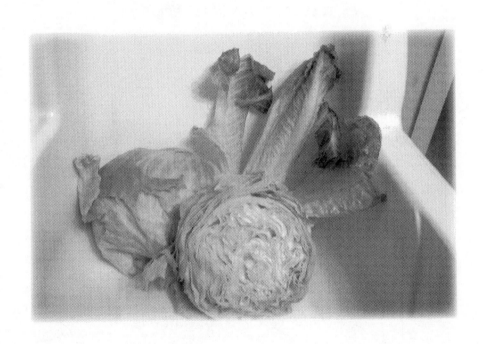

"Eat your lettuce. Yum, yum, yum;

Lettuce surely is yum, yum, yum;

Lettuce is crispy and delicious;

Lettuce surely is good for you.

Vitamins and Minerals are good for you;

Good for your eyes, cells, brains, bones and skin;

Good for your heart, blood and high fiber too.

Eat lettuce daily. Yum, yum, yum!"

They cheered and cheered and cheered just to have her try. Chelsea shut her eyes, pretending to fall asleep.

"No thank you! It's not that one.

Try once more. It's not that one."

They thought and thought and thought and then finally made a decision; and it was Zucchini

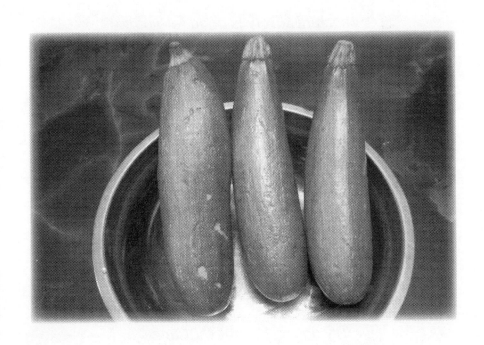

"Eat Zucchini. Yum, yum, yum;

Zucchini surely is yum, yum, yum;

Zucchini is mushy and delicious;

Zucchini surely is good for you.

Vitamins and Minerals are good for you;

Good for your eyes, cells, joints and skin;

Good for your heart, liver, tummy and fiber too.

Eat your Zucchini daily. Yum, yum, yum!"

They cheered and cheered and cheered and cheered. Guess what! Chelsea still shook her head because they couldn't guess it right.

"No thank you! It's not that one.

Try again. It's not that one."

Sabella became very hungry and tired and needed some rest; but changed her mind and pushed herself. They thought and thought and it was Peas.

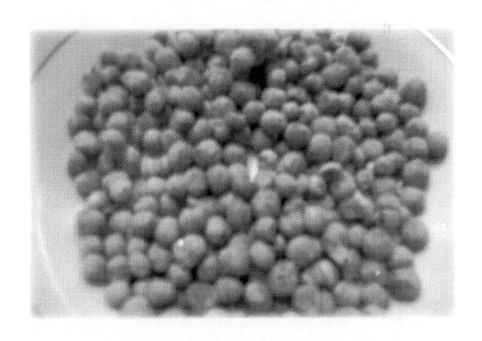

"Eat your peas. Yum, yum, yum;

Peas surely are yum, yum, yum;

Peas are mushy and delicious;

Peas surely are good for you.

Vitamins and Minerals are good for you;

Good for your eyes, cells, blood, brains, bones and skin;

Good for your heart, tummy, weight, joints and smiles too.

Eat peas daily, they are yum, yum, yum!"

They chanted and cheered away but Chelsea shook her head no, no, no.

"No thank you! It's not that one.

You may try again. It's not that one."

They made another guess and it was Melon.

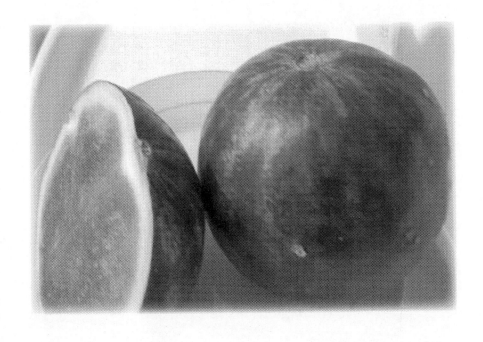

"Eat your melons. Yum, yum, yum;

Melons surely are yum, yum, yum;

Melons are juicy and delicious;

Melons surely are good for you.

Vitamins and Minerals are good for you;

Good for your eyes, cells, lungs, kidneys and bones;

Good for your heart, blood, muscles and fiber too.

Eat melons daily, they are yum, yum, yum!"

They cheered and chanted to have her try but Chelsea shook her head no, no, no.

"No thank you! It's not that one.

Try again. It's not that one."

They made another decision and it was Plum.

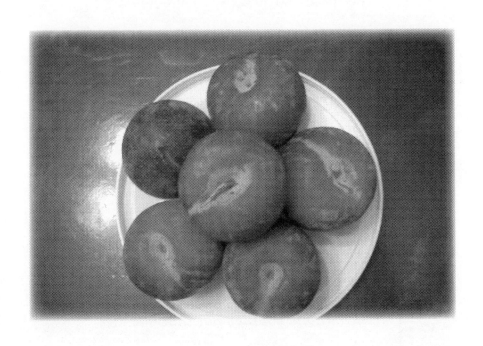

"Eat your Plum. Yum, yum, yum;

Plums surely are yum, yum, yum;

Plums are juicy and delicious;

Plums surely are good for you.

Vitamins and Minerals are good for you;

Good for your eyes, cells, blood, brains and bones;

Good for your heart, soothes colds and flu.

Eat plums daily, yum, yum, yum!"

They chanted to have her try but Chelsea still shook her head meaning no, no, no.

"No thank you! It's not that one.

Try another one. It's not that one."

They made a decision and it was Berries.

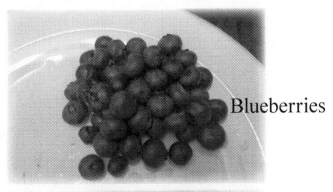

Blueberries

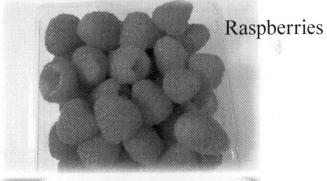

Raspberries

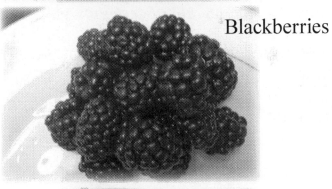

Blackberries

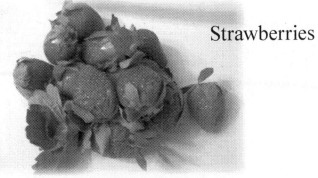

Strawberries

"Eat your Berries. Yum, yum, yum;

Berries surely are yum, yum, yum;

Berries are juicy and delicious;

Berries surely are good for you.

Vitamins and Minerals are good for you;

Good for the eyes, cells, liver, tummy, brains and skin.

Good for your heart, weight, make you smile and fiber too.

Eat your berries daily. Berries are yum, yum, yum!"

They cheered and pleaded to have her try but Chelsea shook her head then chuckled and chuckled and chuckled.

"No thank you! It's not that one.

Try again. It's not that one."

They paused to take a look at what was left that they were missing and then made a guess and it was Squash.

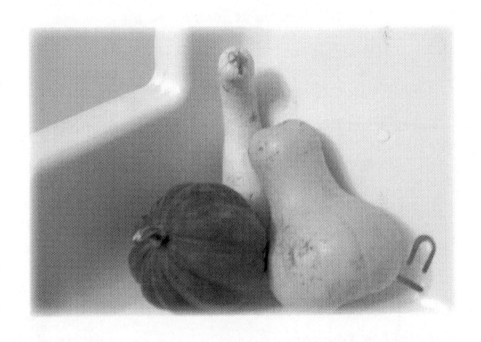

"Eat your squash. Yum, yum, yum;

Squash surely is yum, yum, yum;

Squash is mushy and delicious;

Squash surely is good for you.

Vitamins and Minerals are good for you;

Good for your eyes, cells, joints, muscles and bones;

Good for your heart, blood, lungs and high fiber too.

Eat squash daily, they are yum, yum, yum!"

They chanted away to have her try but Chelsea shook her head again and again.

"No thank you! It's not that one

Try yet again. It's not that one."

Sabella became more and more hungry and tired then finally decided to get some rest, leaving Chelsea's mum to plead, chant and cheer alone. She thought and thought and it was Sweet Potatoes.

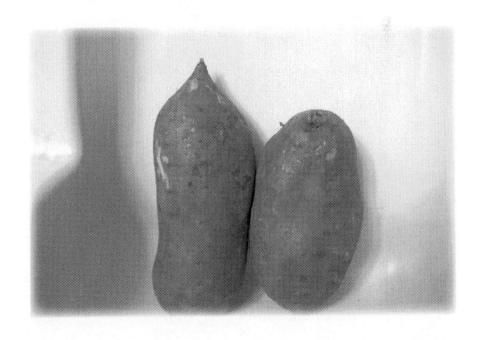

"Eat sweet potatoes. Yum, yum, yum;

Sweet Potatoes surely are yum, yum, yum;

Sweet Potatoes are mushy and delicious;

Sweet Potatoes surely are good for you.

Vitamins and Minerals are good for you;

Good for the eyes, cells, kidneys, muscles, bones and skin;

Good for your heart, blood, tummy, teeth and fiber too.

Eat Sweet Potatoes. Yum, yum, yum!"

Her mother chanted and chanted to have her try but Chelsea shook her head again and again.

"No thank you! It's not that one.

Try again. It's not that one."

Mother thought again; and it was Grapes.

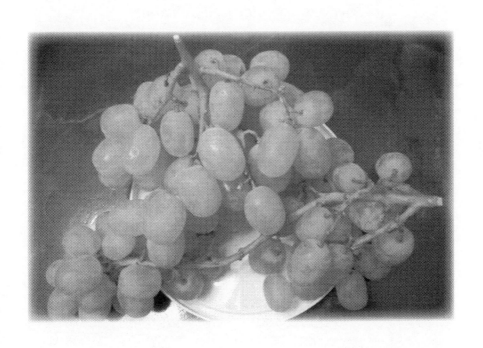

"Eat your grapes. Yum, yum, yum;

Grapes surely are yum, yum, yum;

Grapes are juicy and delicious;

Grapes surely are good for you.

Vitamins and Minerals are good for you;

Good for your eyes, cells, kidneys and brains;

Good for your heart, tummy and lungs.

Eat your grapes daily, they are yum, yum, yum!"

Mother, hungry and exhausted managed to have her try but Chelsea still shook her head no, no, no.

"No thank you! It's not that one.

Try again. It's not that one."

Mother looked around to see what was left and it was Kiwifruit.

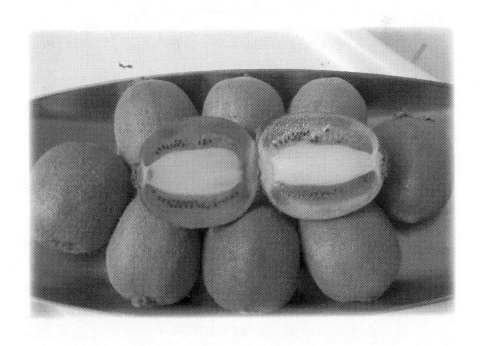

"Eat your kiwi fruit. Yum, yum, yum;

Kiwi fruit surely is yum, yum, yum;

Kiwi fruit is juicy and delicious;

Kiwi fruit surely is good for you.

Vitamins and Minerals are good for you;

Good for your eyes, hair, lungs and skin;

Good for your heart, nails, teeth and fiber too.

Eat your kiwi daily. They are yum, yum, yum!"

Mother managed to cheer to have her try. Chelsea shook her head from left to right.

"No thank you! It's not that one.

Please try again. It's not that one."

Mother was very v-e-r-y hungry but didn't want to quit. She made another guess and this time; it was Asparagus.

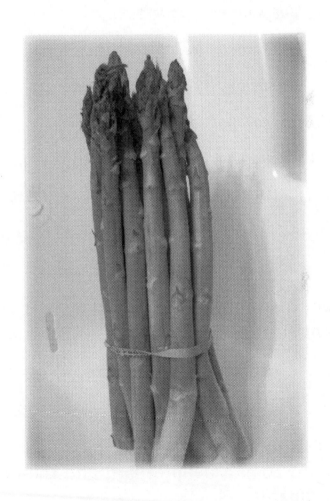

"Eat your asparagus. Yum, yum, yum;

Asparagus surely is yum, yum, yum;

Asparagus is crunchy and delicious;

Asparagus surely is good for you.

Vitamins and Minerals are good for you;

Good for your eyes, cells, brains, bones and skin;

Good for the heart, makes you smile and fiber too.

Eat asparagus daily. Yum, yum, yum!"

Mother crossed her fingers, hoping that was it; but Chelsea shook her head from side to side.

"No thank you! It's not that one.

Try again. It's not that one."

Mother d-r-a-g-g-e-d herself to plead, chant and cheer. She took a deep breath and then chose Pomegranates.

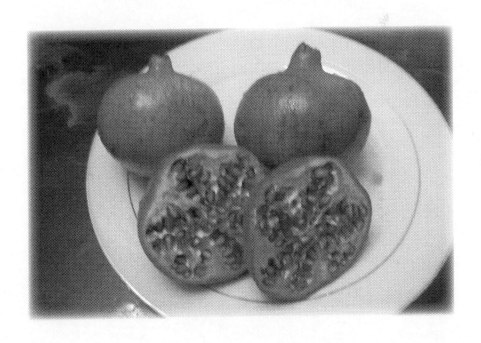

"Eat pomegranates. Yum, yum, yum;

Pomegranates surely are yum, yum, yum;

Pomegranates are juicy and delicious;

Pomegranates surely are good for you.

Vitamins and Minerals are good for you;

Good for your cells, blood vessels, bones and brains;

Good for your heart. Make you smile too.

Eat Pomegranates daily. Yum, yum, yum!"

Her mother pleaded, chanted and cheered to have her try but Chelsea shook her head again and again.

"No thank you! It's not that one.

Try again. It's not that one."

Mother was very tired and hungry. She wanted to rest but changed her mind. Then it was Oranges.

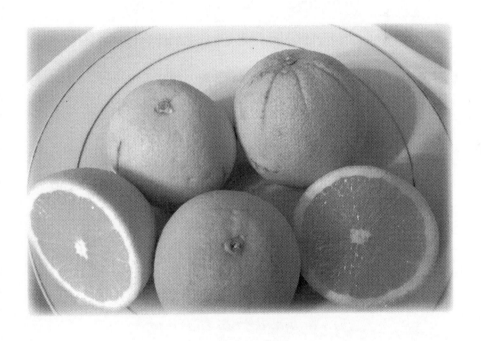

"Eat your Oranges. Yum, yum, yum;

Oranges surely are yum, yum, yum;

Oranges are juicy and delicious;

Oranges surely are good for you.

Vitamins and Minerals are good for you;

Good for your eyes, cells, blood, tummy and skin.

Good for your heart, kidneys, teeth, bones and fiber too.

Eat oranges daily, they are yum, yum, yum!"

Mother managed to have her try but Chelsea shook her head no, no, no.

"No thank you! It's not that one.

Try again. It's not that one."

Mrs. Emeka was almost giving up. She looked around to see what was left and then prayed and prayed to have it be; and it was Parsnips.

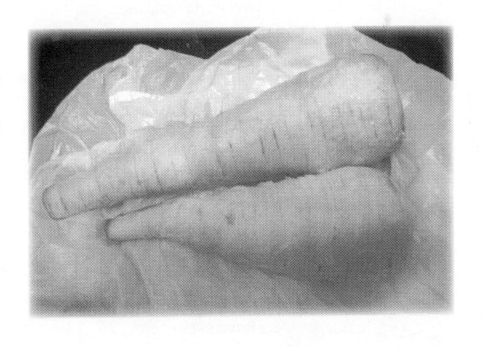

"Eat your Parsnips. Yum, yum, yum;

Parsnips surely are yum, yum, yum;

Parsnips are crunchy and delicious;

Parsnips surely are good for you.

Vitamins and Minerals are good for you;

Good for your cells, blood, bones and fiber too;

Good for your heart, tummy, teeth and gums.

Eat your parsnips daily, they are yum, yum, yum!"

Mother cheered to have her try. Chelsea jumped from her seat then up and down:

"Yes please, that is the one.

You got me. I have to try one."

The rest joined in to watch her try. Chelsea managed and managed to try parsnip salad. She took a tiny bite; then another and yet another.

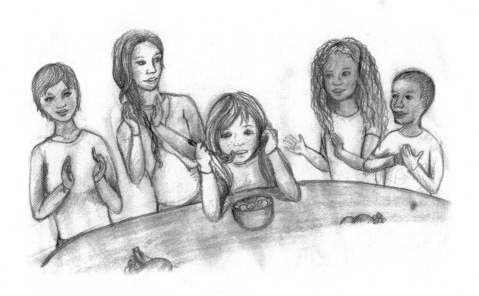

"Fruits and Vegetables taste so good;

Parsnip salad tastes so good; I will taste all food."

Chelsea tasted and tasted and tasted them all. Guess what? She liked them all. They all clapped and cheered then happily ate their meals.

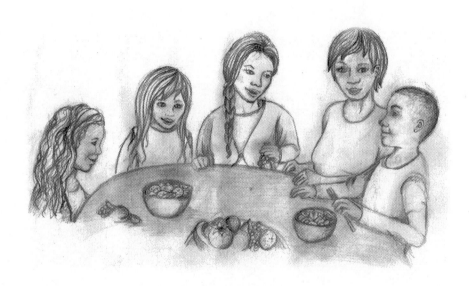

Vegetable party did it all. These children love to eat their Fruits and Vegetables. What about you? Uhmmm!

The end!

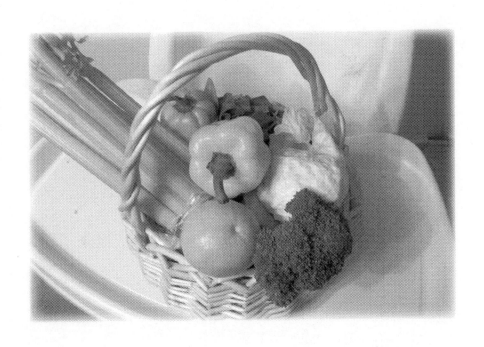

Author's Biography

Philomina Uzoamaka Emeka-Iheukwu was born in Nigeria on the 22nd May, 1978. She has longed to become a writer from a very young age. Her deep desire to write made her study Journalism from the Institute of Management and Technology, Enugu, and then proceeded to the University of Nigeria, Enugu for a Post Graduate Degree and a Master's Degree in Public Relations.

Her love for children drove her to write fiction stories to help little-people (children) cope and overcome real life challenges in a very fun way.

Besides writing stories, she also loves to write healthy recipes, cooking, exercising, dancing, playing and reading to her children. She has also authored a very healthy cookbook, *Cook Healthy, Eat Healthy, Feel Healthy America*. This is her first children's book. Presently, she resides in Rochester, New York with her husband of many years and their beautiful children.

Contact her at:
philominaemekaiheukwu@yahoo.com

Acknowledgements

For support and encouragement, I would like to thank my husband, Sylvester Iheukwu, Onyinye Emeka, Mum and especially Frank Martello of Countertop Creations and his members of staff.

For her close reading to make this manuscript better, Chris Pittaway and especially Rachel Farley for her illustrations.

For every single thing, glory to God!